Low Carb Diet

The Practical Guide to Enjoy Your

Family Meals Living a Low Carb Lifestyle

Natalie Bennett

Table of Contents

Chapter 1

Why Is the Population Becoming Fat?

Weight gain and obesity have become causes of health concerns in the western world. Obesity is one of the leading causes of preventable death in the world today. Studies have been conducted to establish the reasons why the world population seems to be gaining weight. Research has shown, for instance, that the general weight of the population today, is much higher than it was in the 1960s.

What are the factors that have contributed to this turn of events and what are the intervention measures that can be instituted to control it? Studies have shown that although our children still engage in physical exercises, just like the children of yester years, they still add weight and, in some cases, get obese. For the older people, lack of exercise, among other issues has been cited a reason for weight gain or becoming fat.

Obesity and weight gain have been attributed to the foods we eat. Research shows that we have increased our food intake which unfortunately contains a higher percentage of sugar than what the world population used to ingest about fifty years ago.

Also, the amount of fat that we eat has considerably increased. This coupled with lack of exercise have been cited as the leading causes of weight gain. It is an established fact that when we get large portions of fatty foods, creamy desserts, alcohol, and soft drinks full of sugar, our calorie intake gets higher.

With a higher calorie intake, we are expected to do a lot of exercises to burn the excess calories. If this is not done, there is a calorie pile up that leads to weight gain. The solution to these problems lies in the ability to change our eating habits. One way of controlling unnecessary weight gain is the eating low carb foods. This way, the number of calories in the food is closely controlled and helps in making one healthier.

Low Carb diets have been defined differently depending on whether the point of discussion is centred on number of calories derived from carbohydrates or the percentage of carbohydrates in a diet. Generally, though, low carb diets can be described as those diets that help the body to derive between 5% to 45 % of calories from Carbohydrates. The normal percentage of calories that is supposed to be derived from Carbohydrates, according to the U.S. guidelines on health is between 50% to 65%.

Therefore, a low carb diet refers to a conscious effort to try and limit the intake of foods with high carbohydrate levels, especially those that cause a significant rise in blood sugar.

Although the debate on the advantages of a low carb diet is still going on, it is true that the tolerance of carbohydrates in the body varies from person to person.

This type of diet, then, will suit or benefit those who are sensitive or whose tolerance to carbohydrates is low. The approach is to encourage the reduction of the intake of carbohydrates to levels that the body can tolerate. This approach targets the reduction or elimination from our diets foods like potatoes, white rice, white flour, and sugar from the diet.

The reduction of carbohydrates intake has been known to cause weight loss in people. To control this, a low carb diet should be closely monitored so that immediately signs of weight loss are noticed; the intake of carbohydrates is slowly increased until the body can control blood glucose.

It is also advisable to embrace the ketogenic diet where the body generates energy from body fats instead of the glucose. This leads the body into what is called fat adaptation or keto adaptation.

This adaptation encourages body metabolism which leads to improvement of stamina. Energy from fat is long lasting unlike energy from glucose which quickly diminishes.

Chapter 2

What Is A Low Carb Diet?

We often hear about low carb diets and how successful they prove to be in losing weight, but what is a low Carb diet exactly? The term "low-carb" means low in carbohydrate. Carbohydrates are usually found in foods like pasta, potatoes, fruit, bread and rice. A low carb diet does not entail any specific diet, nor does it include well-defined steps to losing weight. It is a rather loose term that varies according to the person who uses it. Some common features though, include consuming foods that are low in carbohydrate and glycaemic. The consumption of carbohydrates leads the body to excrete insulin.

As carbohydrates get digested, glucose - effect of insulin excretion- either gets burned by our body if it we need immediate energy or else gets stored as fat. More seriously, after consuming a meal that consists mainly of carbohydrates, the level of insulin in our body goes suddenly up and after a short time suddenly down. This effect causes us to be hungry only after 2 or 4 hours from our last meal, leading us to a vicious circle of being hungry, then eating and finally storing fat.

The main ways to define a low carb diet, following the initial question "What Is A Low Carb Diet?", is to clarify whether you are talking about the actual carbohydrate that an adult consumes daily or about the percentage of the calories in a person's diet that comes from carbohydrates. The usual number of calories that are allowed in an adult's diet is about 50-60%. So, any percentage of calories coming from carbohydrates that is below that, can be thought of as low carb. The most common misconception about low carb diets is that people who follow this kind of eating plan are striving to consume a zero amount of carb.

That is not only untrue, but it is also near to impossible considering carbohydrates are hidden in most of the food we consume, especially processed food. A diet low in carbs, as the name itself demonstrates, tries to reduce the carbohydrates in a low level, not eliminate them completely.

Another common myth is that a low carb diet forbids you from eating fruits and vegetables. The truth is that this food category is rich in carbohydrate, but that does not mean one should eliminate them from their diet. Fruits and veggies are the carbohydrates one should consume in a diet that is low of, but not deprived of carbs. Among the benefits one could gain from following a low carb diet, is first and foremost the loss of weight and the increase of energy. People find themselves to be less sleepy, have better concentration and some cases have shown that people are experiencing a better mood. Bad thoughts and feelings seem to be seriously reduced or lifted away. One cannot overstate the beneficial results of low carb eating habits.

People have noticed improvements in their metabolism, a benefit that is a kick start for a diet focused on losing weight, even if the weight loss is initially insignificant. A shift in the metabolism is indispensable on the road to a healthy way of life and weight loss process.

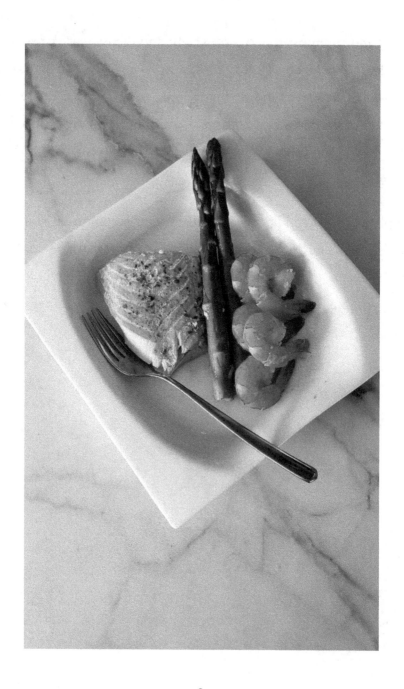

Chapter 3

The Benefits of a Low Carb Diet

When you choose a diet, you want to make sure there are plenty of positive benefits beyond losing weight. You want to be healthier overall by eating in the manner the diet instructs you to eat daily. You also want to be able to follow the plan for life instead of just a few weeks or months. The benefits of a low carb diet will provide the healthy daily plan you can implement for life.

You may not realize that eating carbs can increase the chance of negative health issues. By reducing the volume of carbs daily that you eat, some medical conditions you often experience may occur less often. The frequency of headaches, joint pain, and trouble concentrating will diminish when you reduce the intake of carbs. This may help you reduce the amount of pain medicine you take when the pain of headaches and joints go away. So, you will feel healthier and save money on medicine by the benefits of a low carb diet.

Often when you diet mood swings can cause the process to be difficult. The highs and lows of mood and energy can cause you to binge eat. Another benefit of the low carb diet is the balancing of mood and energy. The body gets more consistent energy from protein and other nutrients than from carbs. Carbs bring on short term energy spurts that will drop your energy level quickly once the carbs are digested. By lowering the volume of carbs, you eat, your energy will come from other nutrients that are more consistent energy reducing mood and energy swings.

If you enjoy exercise and want to tone and build muscle tissue which helps fight fat in your body, a low carb diet can help. After a workout, your muscles are very sensitive to insulin and do not need as many carbs as some people may think. By eating a low carb diet, your muscles after a workout will draw in more amino acids from your meal. The amino acids will help the muscles heal from the workout quicker and burn more fat.

The impact or prevention of diabetes can be helped by a low carb diet. If you have diabetes a low carb diet may help balance your insulin level more throughout the day. If you have family members with diabetes and want to avoid getting the disease yourself, a low carb diet is a good healthy way to naturally balance your insulin.

So, as you can see, there are many benefits to a low carb diet beyond just losing weight. You will see an improvement in your weight, but you will also have more energy and feel healthier. That is the goal of losing weight as well; to be healthier.

Eating more vegetables and proteins as well as fruits and nuts can be a good start to a low carb diet. Gradually reduce your intake of breads, sweets, and items made from white flour and white sugar. You can find many low carb diet recipes for free on blogs, websites, and food preparing television shows.

Chapter 4

Are Low Carb Diets Safe?

Obesity must be the most widely spread issue worldwide irrespective of demographic or the geographic differences. It has gained so much attention lately that the concept of weight loss has opened thousands of lucrative business opportunities. Ironically, this commercialization seems to have a negative impact on actual weight loss.

Calorie intake and burning calories, the two main variables of the weight loss equation have been exaggerated so much in the commercial world that in some cases some weight loss programs are a threat to good health. Low carb diet came into the existence as a solution for maintaining the calorie intake variable in precise levels. How it helps you to lose weight is simple logic.

Once the intake drops the body starts to make use of the stored fat which leads to weight loss. Of course, it will lead to weight loss, but will it be a safe process? The answer is not a simple yes or a no. Even though weight loss gurus emphasize importance repeatedly nutritionists and medical community bear a different opinion.

The established opinion is that no matter how effective the results are unless cutting the carbohydrates are done at moderate levels the side effects will lead to disorders in bodily functions. Not only moderate but also it has to be properly chosen.

For example, if you reduce the fat intake without paying attention to the type of fat it might even lead to elevated blood cholesterol levels. You should have the adequate knowledge to determine what should be included and what should not be.

Here according to the example, a properly designed diet plan would have included polyunsaturated fats and mono-unsaturated fats which are considered safe. Same theory applies to all the nutrients just like to fats. Some diet plans even advise to refrain from fruits and vegetables. Such plans do more harm than good. A restriction on fruits like banana or watermelon that have a high glycaemic level might at least have logic to support it. But limiting all the fruits and vegetables is a baseless advice that will deteriorate your health. Reduced intake of calcium rich food like whole grain could even cause serious conditions like osteoporosis. Women with calcium deficiencies tend to suffer from menstrual issues. Most low carb diet plans focus more on protein intake.

Unnecessary amounts of protein make the kidneys work harder to remove excess waste produced by proteins.

Accumulation of harmful waste products might cause kidney stones. Most importantly before selecting a diet plan one should understand his or her body well. A kidney patient should pay attention to the proteins while a heart patient should concentrate more on the fats.

Likewise, there are numerous factors that should be considered before following a low carb diet. Changes in your lifestyle will require changes in diet plans too.

If you start working out or bodybuilding the energy demand of the body is different from what it used to be. Or if you got pregnant changes should come immediately. In cases like these consulting a professional is a must. Extremely "low carb" diets might not be safe. But make them "correct carb" diets and get the lean body you always dreamed while being in good health.

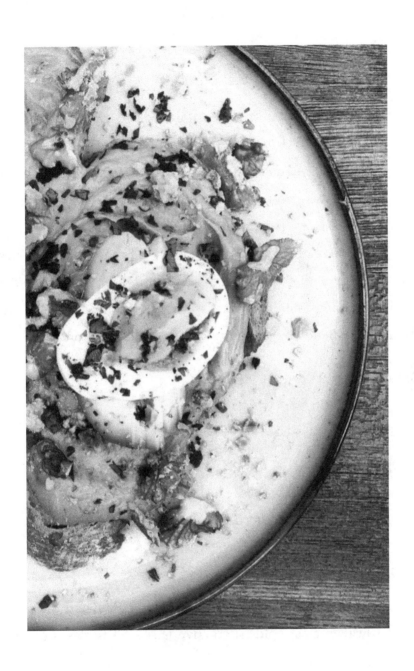

Chapter 5

A Low Carb Sample Meal Plan

While there is an endless supply of different variations to a low carb diet plan one can find and learn about online, it is imperative to at least start off knowing a few basic meal plan ideas to kick start your low carb dieting efforts. So, while the following meal plan ideas are enough to start off with, it is important to note that as with anything "variety is the spice of life" So make sure to learn about and expand your low carb dieting meal variations.

Breakfast

Option 1:

7 Egg White Omelet – allow 2 yolks only

1 cup veges eg. Mushrooms/capsicums

2 Plain Corn Thins (as alternative to bread)

Option 2:

1 cup Oats (cooked 2 cups) – (place ½ cup water in oats then cook in microwave or eat cold (alternative is special K flakes or plain muesli with no dried fruit)

1 heaped tablespoon Natural Pineapple or 2 Kiwi fruit or ½ cup frozen berries

Lunch

Option 1:

3 hard-boiled eggs
A large green leaf salad of your choice
2 Tablespoons of low carb commercial or homemade dressing

Optional: Sprinkle with Spicy Sweet Pecans

Option 2:

200g Cooked Lean Meat: chicken breast, Fish of any kind, Rump

Steak, Eggs (10 egg white) (230g raw)

1 full cup greens (coleslaw, herbslaw packs at supermarkets, frozen vege is fine)

Tablespoon of lite oil dressing (Italian, french or olive oil)

1 full cup Basmati Rice (1 cup raw = 1.5 cup cooked). Or medium sweet potato (fist size)

Afternoon Snack

Option 1:

1 oz string cheese

Option 2:

20 Plain Nuts = cashews/almonds or walnuts (inside palm size)

Dinner

Option 1:

6 Egg Omlette with 6 slices smoked salmon with salad on side

Option 2:

200g Grilled Chicken

2 full cup greens (coleslaw packs as mentioned)

2 Tablespoon Lite Cottage Cheese – OPTIONAL

Dessert

Option 1:

8-10 strawberries, dipped in

¼ cup sugar-free chocolate sauce (ganache)

Option 2:

½ cup of low sugar jell-o

Chapter 6

Shopping Advice for Low Carb Dieters

Watching carbs to lose weight, or stay healthy, should not cost you a fortune. Which is why including high-priced foods in your diet is not necessary, for sure.

There are countless less costly, yet delicious, options that are low in carbs. So, let's get started saving money on the most delicious, low carb foods. First things first; we all know packaged food is costly. Swap it out with home-cooked dishes made from tender meat and fresh vegetables. Pre-packaged junk foods will only drain money off your wallet while it will not do good to your waistline, either.

You, next, might want to consider purchasing food in season. Of course, would not you dress heavily in winter, and lightly in summer? Likewise, you would like to order fruits and veggies when they are in season - that is when they are cheapest.

Otherwise, it costs a lot more when produce is flown in from other countries. But by purchasing in-season vegetables, even freezing them, you can get yourself your favourites year-round, yet cheaply.

It is also possible to spend less on meat. While the expensive beef tenderloin is a tasty cut of meat, the chuck and sirloin cuts make a delicious taste at a much-reduced price. They contain streaks of fat running throughout the meat, a thing that makes them tender, juicer and super delicious. They are best suitable to slow cooking - no wonder you should think soups, stews, braises and roasts. In the same respect, protein that is priced right helps stretch your dollar, as well. There is more to controlling carbs than meat - do not fall into a supper slump. Break the monotony of your dinner meat by including some eggs. Besides, you can prepare them in any way you like poached, scrambled, omelette, crustless quiche, etc. Moreover, tofu and other soy foods could replace the usual sources of chicken and turkey protein yet give you a variety of nutrients.

You can save on snacks, too. Get low-carb snacks, including shakes and nutrition bars, cheaply at store specials. Buy in bulk. Understand websites that offer items that you regard as your favourites and sign up for their newsletters to catch a heads up on sales.

Do not fail to check for coupons in newspapers circulars, as well. Furthermore, make dishes that can serve double recipes, so you can have dinner for one or two other nights. Likewise, make meals that can serve double duty, like lunch the next day.

Use your low carb leftovers to stretch your dollar. And perhaps you have of this before: planning. But by planning your recipes and meals for the week, you help make yourself prepared, always. You will not have to take that extra trip to the vending machine, or order take-out for your dinner. Wait, do you want to get all that that junk in your tummy?

Among other things, get to know some smart shopping strategies. Regarding pork, for instance, get less costly cuts like shoulder and rib chops, which should be tastier when well prepared. Also, purchasing whole chicken should see you save some bucks. I hope the tips help you save while you shop delicious, low carb foods.

Like I said, a low carb diet should not cost a fortune. Happy shopping!

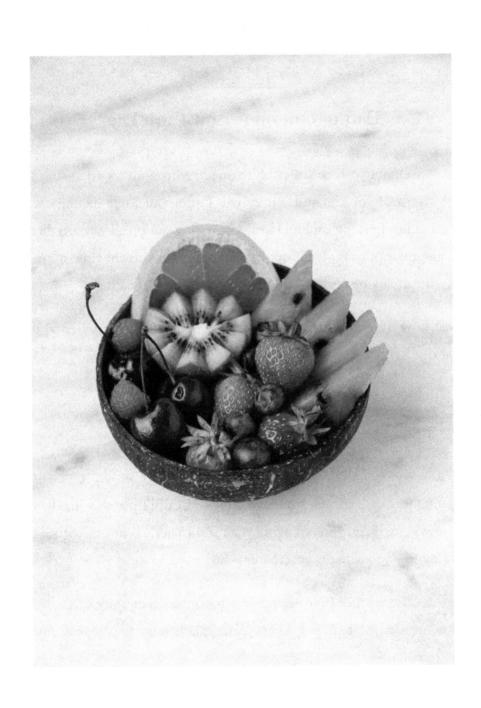

Chapter 7

Eating Out on A Low Carb Die

Dieting can be stressful if you are constantly worried about which foods you can and cannot eat. Eating out while dieting can sometimes be a nightmare. However, eating out on a low carb diet is just the opposite. It is very easy to adapt food from almost any cuisine at any restaurant to suit a low carb way of eating.

Just remembering three things will keep you on track when you eat out:

1. Know what you can eat, and what to avoid!

2. Plan ahead!

3. Stick to your guns!

Eating low carb means you have a lot of flexibility with your diet. Knowing which foods to avoid makes it easier to eat out without trying to guess what is acceptable.

Great choices to look for when eating out include meats that are not breaded or battered, vegetables, salads, and fish that is not battered.

Potatoes are generally off the menu, but why not try extra veggies instead? Consider eating 'outside the box'. If you want a juicy burger, go ahead and have it, without the bun. Replace the fries with carrot sticks to round out your meal. Salads offer unlimited options, as almost any meats and vegetables can be thrown in, and many restaurants offer some type of salad on their menu. Steak and mixed vegetables are always a great choice, and tasty, too!

Perhaps the most overlooked key to successfully eating out on a low carb diet is planning. This simple step can save a lot of stress and worry. You will already know what you can eat, so the next step is finding out what is on offer at the place you want to eat at.

Go online to view menus ahead of time. You can even call restaurant and ask questions about food preparation, ingredients. This way, you will be armed with the info needed to make good food choices. This step eliminates the stress and worry over what you will order once you arrive, so you will be able to focus on enjoying your meal!

The most important thing you can do when eating out low carb is to stick to it. Many are tempted by the breadbasket, teased by the desert tray, and give in to the pressure to be 'normal'. Maybe you do not want to seem demanding.

Whatever the reason, just remember, you deserve to feel healthy and be happy. If it helps, consider your low carb diet the same as anyone that requires a special diet for a medical condition. There will be some foods you just cannot eat, but do not be afraid to ask for the ones you can!

With more people choosing to eat low carb, restaurants are adjusting many of their menu items to accommodate. There are lots of great options available if you want to eat out and enjoy low carb foods. Knowing what you can eat, planning, and sticking to it will keep you on track with your low carb diet. Use these simple steps to enjoy eating out on a low carb diet anytime!

Chapter 8

Maintaining A Low Carb Diet

One great advantage of a low-carb diet is the fact that you will not have to worry about the number of calories you take. Furthermore, you will not have to keep count and track of your calories. This is because maintaining a low carb lifestyle is all about the amount of carbohydrate you take in your food. With this kind of diet, you need to have a plan that suggests the amount of carbohydrate you need to take in a day.

This plan will also contain other food nutrients you should take to complement your diet. The idea is to decrease your carbohydrate intake and to be able to reduce your sugar and insulin levels. Your body will then have to burn the stored fat in your body making you lose weight. To create the best diet to help you in maintaining a low carb lifestyle, you need to be aware of five simple and easy to do tips.

These are suggestions to help you make the most out of your diet. This way, you can be sure to get the effective weight lose results.

First, you need to have your health assessed by your doctor. This is the initial step you need to take before you decide to undertake your dieting plan. Consulting your physician is a good way to establish the best food types to include in your diet. The doctor will help you know what food to refrain from and get suggestions on how to plan your diet menu.

Secondly, you must have an objective for maintaining a low-carb lifestyle. The goal of any diet low in carbohydrate is to lose weight. Establishing your main goal will help you fit your diet into your lifestyle. Here, you will know what nutritional foods to introduce into your diet; one that leads to successfully achieving your long-term weight lose goal.

Thirdly, for your diet plan to work you need motivation to follow through with your plan even when faced with temptations. You need to find a way to remind yourself of your goal. Thinking about how you will feel or look when you are slimmer is a good incentive.

Additionally, you need to tune your attitude, be positive and believe you can achieve your weight loss objective.

Besides, monitor the amount of food you take and take weight often to find out how you are doing. It is best you have a journal where you can record your findings. This journal will help you find out whether your diet plan is successful or not.

Lastly, after all has been said and done you will have to be patient and be consistent in your dieting. Maintaining a low carb diet is not very easy. However, you will be successful if you maintain your plan and make it a habit. With time, it will become a lifestyle and part of you.

Like any dieting plan, you may fall off track occasionally. However, you should get back up and continue with your plan. From time to time, you may have to consult your doctor to ensure you do not have health complications and to ensure your diet is working effectively.

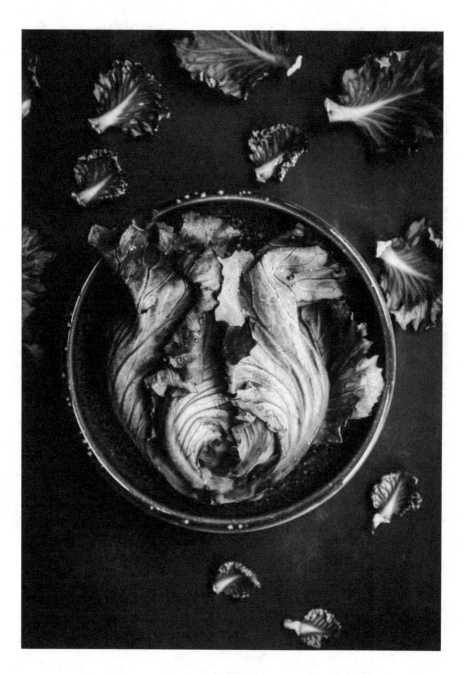

Chapter 9

Common Mistakes on A Low

Carb Diet One does not have to attend a class to know about the common mistakes on a low Carb diet. Carb as it is referred in this context refers to food nutrient (carbohydrate) present in foods like potatoes, bread, pun cakes etc. The following are the common mistakes about low cab diet.

Getting wrong information - Some individuals assume that eating low Carb diet simply means eating meat every day. This is wrong; everybody requires knowledge on how to reduce carbohydrates, the foods that have carbohydrates and eating a low carb diet.

Surrendering in the middle of the process - There are a variety of approaches to low carb dieting and there are problems at the beginning. It is important to figure out which approach is good for you to avoid giving up in the middle of the process. Some of the complication that arises for example Carb crash scares a lot of people hence they back down at the beginning.

Lack of sufficient fat This could be mistaken for a low carb diet because of thinking that low carb means low fat. At the start, people can manage low fat dieting but as time goes this will lead to them using up their own body fat hence getting hungry very fast. Therefore, it is important to add fat to your body while on low carb diet.

Lack of enough vegetables in the diet - While dieting on low Carb diet some people tend to forget including vegetables and fruits in their diet. This will be disastrous in the end because vegetables and fruits should be eaten in large quantities by one dieting on low carb especially fruits that are low in sugar.

Too much eating - It is of no use to count the number of calories in a low carb diet. This does not mean that one must keep on eating and eating just because he or she is eating foods that are low in carb. You are advised to only eat when one is hungry and stop when satisfied.

Poor planning - Sticking in a new eating programme sometimes might be a problem and one might find himself or herself doing what they used to do before. Therefore, one is advised to plan before hand to facilitate free adoption of the new eating habit which means you will know what to eat and when to eat what.

Use of low carb packaged foods - When buying low carb foods are packaged it is of great importance to understand ingredients.

Most of them contain maltitol which is bad sugar that is not required by a lot of bodies. Therefore, this packaged low carb foods need to undergo careful experiments.

Lack of variety - Most people might find limited variety of foods that are low carb yet there are plenty, the only thing to avoid in low cab diet is sugar and starch. Every cuisine in the planet has a low carb variety; also, most dishes can be decarded.

Insufficient fibre in the diet - Eating of vegetables and fruits help in ensuring that one eats enough quantities of fibre. But forgetting or skipping to eat vegetables and fruits reduces the level of fibre intake in the body and this can be disastrous in the long run.

30 Low Carb Recipes

APPETIZERS

Lobster Salad in Endive

Makes 24 appetizers; serves 6 to 8

If you want to be good to yourself and your guests at the same time, ask your fish store to sell you cooked fresh lobster meat, instead of cooking a lobster yourself. This is a great summer appetizer or a special treat for New Year's Eve.

This recipe is also good, and not quite so expensive, with cooked shrimp or crabmeat. You will see that a little salad makes a lot of appetizers.

Ingredients

- ❖ 3/4-pound fresh cooked lobster meat, small-diced
- ❖ 1/2 cup good mayonnaise
- ❖ 1/2 cup small-diced celery (1 stalk)
- ❖ 1 tablespoon capers, drained
- ❖ 11/2 tablespoons minced fresh dill

- ❖ Pinch kosher salt
- ❖ Pinch freshly ground black pepper
- ❖ 4 heads Belgian endive

Direction

Combine the lobster, mayonnaise, celery, capers, dill, salt, and pepper. With a sharp knife, cut off the base of the endive and separate the leaves. Use a teaspoon to fill the end of each endive leaf with lobster salad. Arrange on a platter and serve.

Connie Wheeler adds, "Make sure you use real lobster though. I was perusing through my carbohydrate counter just yesterday at fish and seafood and noticed that the fake lobster or crab is high in carbohydrates at 8.5 carbs per 3 oz.

Hot Artichoke and Spinach Dip

Ingredients

- ❖ 1 pkg. Cream Cheese
- ❖ 1 can 14 oz. Progresso Artichoke Hearts, drained, coarsely chopped
- ❖ 1/2 cup Spinach, frozen chopped, or steamed
- ❖ 1/4 cup Mayonnaise (do not use Miracle Whip)
- ❖ 1/4 cup Parmesan Cheese
- ❖ 1/4 cup Romano Cheese (You can use all Parmesan)
- ❖ 1 clove garlic, finely minced
- ❖ 1/2 tsp. fresh basil (dry 1 tbsp. Basil)
- ❖ 1/4 cup Mozzarella Cheese grated
- ❖ 1/4 tsp. Garlic Salt
- ❖ Salt and Pepper to taste

Direction

Allow cream cheese to come to room temperature.

Cream together mayonnaise, Parmesan, Romano cheese, garlic, basil, and garlic salt. Mix well.

Add the artichoke hearts and spinach (careful to drain this well) and mix until blended. Store in a container until you are ready to use.

Spray pie pan with Pam, pour in dip, and top with cheese. Bake at 350 degrees for 25 minutes or until the top is browned. Serve with cucumber slices, pork rinds or sliced celery).

Guacamole Dip or Salad Dressing

Ingredients

- ❖ 3 ripe avocados
- ❖ 3 Tbsp. lemon juice
- ❖ 1 small onion very fine chopped
- ❖ 1 tsp. garlic powder
- ❖ 2 Tbsp. mayonnaise
- ❖ Salt and pepper to taste
- ❖ Dash of Tabasco sauce
- ❖ Dash of Worcestershire sauce
- ❖ Very finely chopped jalapenos peppers to taste
- ❖ 1 chopped ripe tomato

Direction

Placed peeled and cut avocados in a medium bowl and on low-speed blend with mixer. Add remaining ingredients, and jalapenos to suit your taste and blend until mixture is thoroughly blended but not soupy. Chill and serve on lettuce as salad or with chips as dip. Place avocado pits in the mixture while being stored in the refrigerator to keep mixture from turning dark.

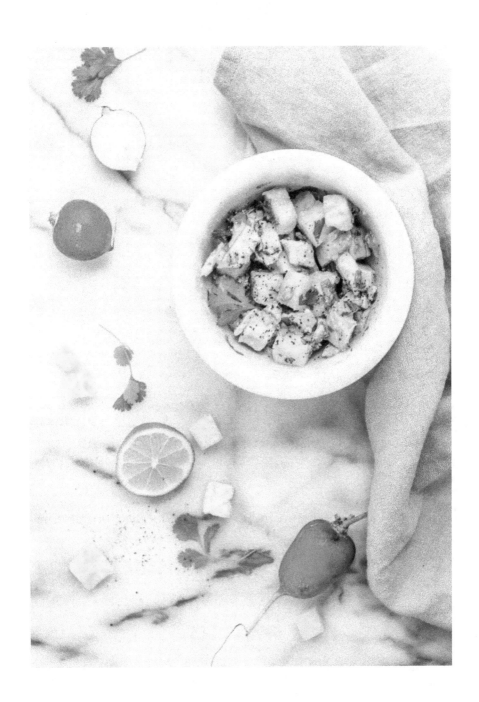

BEVERAGES

Chocolate Shake

Put in blender:

Ingredients

- ❖ 1/4 cup cream
- ❖ 1/4 cup cottage cheese
- ❖ 1/4 cup egg substitute
- ❖ 1/2 cup water
- ❖ 1 Tbsp. cocoa
- ❖ 2 heaping Tbsp. Equal or Splenda
- ❖ 2 heaping Tbsp. lowcarb protein powder (optional)

Blend a few minutes then blend in about 8 cubes ice, one at time.

Hot Chocolate

Ingredients

- ❖ 1 tsp. cocoa powder
- ❖ 2 tsp. Splenda
- ❖ 8 oz hot water.
- ❖ 1 tsp. instant coffee

Mix and enjoy!

Frappachino

Brew 4 cups strong coffee. (make expresso if you like. I use a French press for a full extraction)

Ingredients

- ❖ Add 1 cup to 1.5 cups cream
- ❖ 15 to 30 drops of liquid sweet n low

Stir then cool. Store in fridge, pour over ice and enjoy.

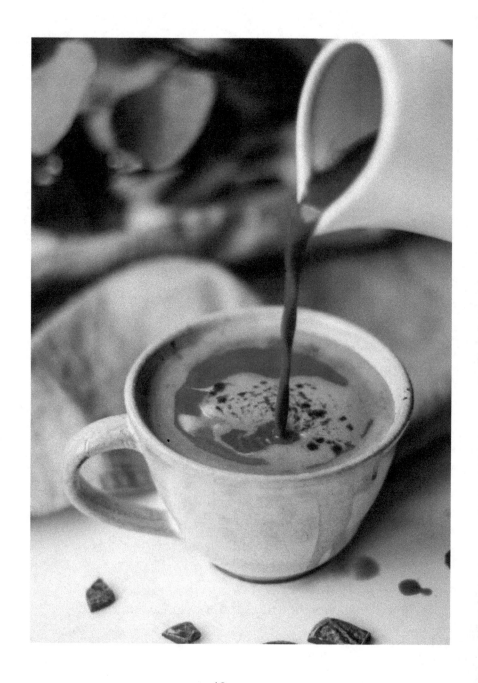

BREADS, SANDWICH, BISCUITS

Low Carb Biscuits

Ingredients

- ❖ 2 cups 12% non-additive, wheat gluten flour from health food store (24 carb grams/cup)
- ❖ 3 tsp. baking powder
- ❖ 1 tsp. salt
- ❖ 1/4 cup shortening
- ❖ 3/8 cup cream
- ❖ 3/8 cup water (combine cream and water to make three quarters cup "milk" substitute)

Direction

Preheat oven to 450. Mix flour, salt and baking powder. Cut in shortening thoroughly – should resemble meal.

Stir in almost all the milk. If dough is not pliable, add just enough milk to make a puffy, easy to roll dough. (Too much milk makes dough sticky, not enough makes biscuits dry - I used all of it).

Make a ball of dough and place on lightly floured surface. Knead 20-25 times or about one-half minute.

Roll out dough to about one-half inch thickness. (Note, it takes a little more effort since gluten is a "binder" - just roll harder).

Cut with a floured cutter (a glass rim will work fine) and place on an ungreased baking sheet. Bake 10-12 minutes or until golden brown. Betty says this makes about 16 1- and 3/4-inch biscuits.

SANDWICH BREAD

Ingredients

- ❖ 1/4 c ground sesame seeds
- ❖ 1/4 c ground flax seeds (0)*
- ❖ 1/4 cup protein powder (2) **
- ❖ 1/4 cup soy flour
- ❖ 3 eggs
- ❖ 1/2 c sour cream
- ❖ 1 1/2 t baking powder
- ❖ 1/2 t salt
- ❖ 4 T olive oil

Direction

Preheat oven 350. Mix all ingredients together. Pour into greased loaf pan. Bake 25 min.

Total: 44 carb, 25 fiber (19 NET carbs), 1563 Calories, 145 fat, 61 protein.

Makes 8 slices @ 2.4 NET carbs, 195 Calories, 18 fat, 8 protein.

*My flax seed package shows 2 carbs, with 2 fiber.

**I used Designer vanilla.

Since this did not rise much, I cut it in half crosswise, then cut each half into 4 slices so they were the size of regular bread. This is better toasted.

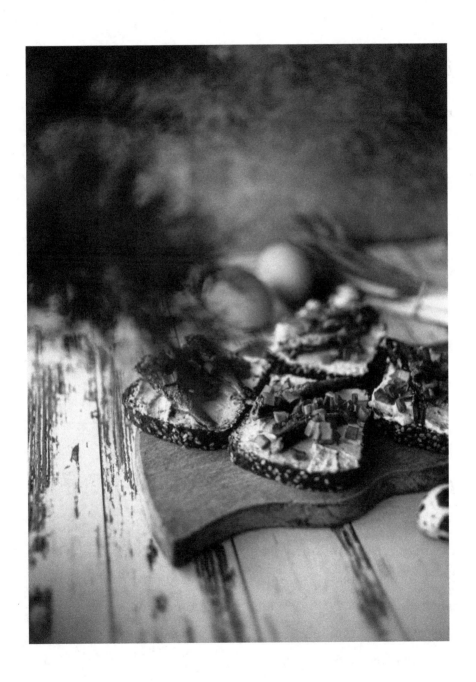

BETTER TASTING PROTEIN BREAD

Ingredients

- ❖ 3/4 cup soy isolate
- ❖ 2 T powdered egg whites
- ❖ 2 pkts Splenda
- ❖ 2 t baking powder
- ❖ dash salt
- ❖ 5 T heavy cream
- ❖ 3 eggs, separated
- ❖ dash cream of tartar
- ❖ 1/4 cup water
- ❖ 1/4 cup oil

<u>Direction</u>

Preheat oven 400 and spray 8" loaf pan. Beat egg whites with cream of tartar until stiff. Mix egg yolks, cream, water and oil. Sift in dry ingredients and mix well with electric mixer. Fold in egg whites carefully. Spoon into prepared pan and smooth top slightly. Bake 25 minutes or till bread pulls away from sides of pan and is nicely browned.

DESSERTS & SWEETS

Egg Custard for 2

Ingredients

- ❖ 1 egg
- ❖ 1 egg yolk
- ❖ 1/2 c. cream mixed with 1/2 cup water
- ❖ 3 tbsp. sugar substitute (Splenda or another heat stable sweetener)
- ❖ 1 tsp. vanilla extract
- ❖ 1/8 tsp. salt
- ❖ 1/8 tsp. ground nutmeg

Direction

Lightly beat the egg and yolk. Add cream, Splenda, vanilla and salt. Pour into two ungreased 6-ounce custard cups

Sprinkle with nutmeg. Set in a pan containing 1/2 to 1 inch of hot water. Bake at 350 degrees for 35 minutes or until set.

Yield: 2 servings. Approx. 5 grams carbohydrate per serving

Chocolate Fudge

Serves 8

Ingredients

- ❖ 2 tablespoons unsweetened cocoa powder
- ❖ 1/2 cup heavy cream
- ❖ 2 tablespoons butter
- ❖ 4 ounces cream cheese
- ❖ 1/2 teaspoon vanilla
- ❖ 3 tablespoons Splenda

Direction

In a small saucepan, over low heat, melt butter. Add heavy cream and cream cheese and whisk until smooth. Add Splenda and adjust for taste. (Add a little more if you need too) Heat until bubbling, stirring constantly. Reduce heat and stir in cocoa and vanilla. Blend well. Pour into a small, buttered dish. Place in the refrigerator to set for 3 to 4 hours. Cut into 8 pieces.

Per Serving: (1 piece) Protein: 1.3g

Carbs: 2.2g / Dietary Fiber: 0.5g

Choice Chocolate

Ingredients

- ❖ 1 oz unsweetened chocolate (the bar kind)
- ❖ 2 tbsp. butter
- ❖ 1 tbsp. cream or sour cream
- ❖ 1 tsp. vanilla extract
- ❖ 8 packets equal
- ❖ 1 oz crushed nuts (macadamias are nice)

Direction

Melt chocolate and butter, carefully. Remove from heat, stir in cream and vanilla, stir in equal, fold in nuts. Pour into tin-foil-lined something or other. Chill Variations on a theme.

* Double the cream and the sweetener. * Or, add 2 tablespoons of peanut butter. * Or pour into mini-muffin tins, then add 1/4 teaspoon PB to each candy. * Or, add 1 teaspoon peppermint extract. * Or, add ANY flavoured extract (raspberry? cherry?) * Or, add twice the amount of mixed nuts w/o crushing for nut clusters.

EGGS & CHEESE

Deluxe Deviled Eggs

Ingredients

- ❖ 6 hard-cooked eggs
- ❖ 1/2 cup sour cream
- ❖ 1/2 cup flaked canned salmon
- ❖ 1/8 teaspoon curry powder
- ❖ 2 teaspoons prepared mustard
- ❖ 2 teaspoons lemon juice
- ❖ 1-1/2 teaspoons Worcestershire sauce
- ❖ Salt, pepper
- ❖ Paprika

Direction

Shell eggs, then cut in halves lengthways and remove yolks. Mash yolks and mix with sour cream, salmon, curry powder, mustard, lemon juice, and Worcestershire and season to taste with salt and pepper. Pile mixture into whites and garnish with Paprika. Makes 12 halves.

Cheese Taco Shells

I simply grate enough cheese to cover the bottom of 5 inch (?) small non-stick frying pan, then I fried the cheese until it was nearly browned on one side, flipped it over (pour off grease as needed) and let it brown nearly as much as the first side. To make the taco shell shape I just used my spatula to bend it half over and laid the spatula in between the 'sides' of the 'shell'.

To make sure it kept its shape I used a metal rack type thing (it used to be top of a small inside grill, but you could probably use a rack that cools cookies).

I turned the cheese shell upside down (it helps it to drain also) and made sure the side were the distance apart I prefer for a shell. They were very flavourful and crunchy yet did not fall apart like normal, carbohydrate laden shells! They were great!

I used sharp cheddar--in a non-stick, small frying pan (5 inch). It takes a while to get it done, first grate or slice your cheese. Let it melt (medium heat) completely and there will be very small bubble appearing on top (like pancakes) - make sure you pour off grease as needed. When the one side is browned, carefully flip, let second side start to brown then bend with spatula and hold into position.

I also let mine cool some upside down on a rack, helps to keep the shape! This does take some time so be patient this stuff is great! YUM!

Julie Germain also suggests cutting up those "cheese shells" and making some "cheese tostitos".

Quiche Lorraine

Serves six

Ingredients

- ❖ ½ pound of bacon, crisply fried and crumbled
- ❖ 1 cup shredded natural Swiss cheese
- ❖ 1/3 cup minced red onion
- ❖ 4 eggs
- ❖ 2 cups whipping cream
- ❖ ¼ tsp. salt
- ❖ ¼ tsp. equivalent of sweetener
- ❖ 1/8 tsp. cayenne pepper

Direction

Heat oven to 425. Sprinkle bacon, cheese and onion in the bottom of a 9-inch pie pan. Beat eggs lightly and beat in remaining ingredients. Pour cream mixture into pie pan. Bake in oven for 15 minutes.

Reduce oven temperature to 300 degrees and bake 30 minutes or longer or until a knife inserted 1 inch from the edge comes out clean. Let stand 10 minutes before cutting. Serve in wedges.

This makes a soft-textured quiche. If a firmer texture is desired, cook an additional 10 minutes.

Total calories - 2,051 Total carbohydrates - 25.7

Per serving - 342 Carbohydrates - 4.3

FISH & SEAFOOD

CRAB BROCCOLI CASSEROLE

Ingredients

- ❖ 2 T butter
- ❖ 1/4 c chpd onion
- ❖ 8 oz crab
- ❖ 1/4 t curry
- ❖ 1/4 c cream & 1/4 c water
- ❖ 2 c cooked broccoli
- ❖ 1 c cheddar
- ❖ xanthan gum (thickener)
- ❖ 1/2 t salt
- ❖ 1 T lemon juice

Direction

Preheat oven 350. Grease 1 qt casserole and put cooked broccoli in bottom. Sprinkle with cheese. Melt butter and sauté onion. Add flour, curry powder and salt.

Gradually stir in cream and water mixture. Cook til thickened (may have to add thickener). Add lemon juice and crab.

Pour over broccoli. Bake 30 min.

Serves 2 @ 8 carb, 3 fiber (5 NET carbs), 561 Calories, 43 fat, 38 protein.

FISHY VOLCANOS

Ingredients

- ❖ 12 oz fish fillets (I used flounder)
- ❖ 6 oz can crab
- ❖ 1/4 c grated zucchini
- ❖ 1 T onion powder
- ❖ 1 oz pork rinds, crushed
- ❖ 1 T mayo
- ❖ 1 T mustard
- ❖ 1/3 c heavy cream
- ❖ 1 T soy protein isolate
- ❖ 1 T parmesan
- ❖ cayenne pepper, paprika

Direction

Preheat oven 325. Spray LARGE muffin tin with non-stick spray. Line 6 cups with fish fillet (or several if fillets are small). In bowl, mix crab, zucchini, onion powder and pork rinds. Add remaining ingredients. Divide mixture among fish lined cups. Sprinkle each with little cayenne and paprika. Bake 30 min.

BROILED FISH W/CHEESE

Ingredients

- ❖ 12 oz flounder
- ❖ 2 T melted butter
- ❖ 1/2 c cheddar, shredded
- ❖ 1 T mustard
- ❖ 1 T ketchup or chili sauce

Direction

Brush fish with melted butter and broil 8-10 min till flaky.

Combine remaining ingredients and spoon onto fish. Broil 2-4 min till cheese bubbly and lightly browned.

Serves 2 @ 1 carb, trace fiber, 379 Calories, 23 fat, 40 protein.

MEAT DISHES

Great Meatloaf

Ingredients

- ❖ 1 lb. ground chuck
- ❖ 1 cup pork rinds
- ❖ 1 egg
- ❖ 1/2 cup heavy cream
- ❖ 2 tbsp. Worcestershire sauce
- ❖ 3/4 cup shredded cheese
- ❖ Salt

Direction

Crunch pork rinds up into crumbs. Put the meat in a microwave-safe baking dish. Add the pork rind crumbs, cream, egg, cheese, Worcestershire sauce. Add salt to taste.

Stir until all ingredients are mixed thoroughly and shape into a loaf. Put into microwave and cook for 14 minutes (or until internal temp rises to 150). Makes 4 large servings - 3 grams carbohydrates/serving.

Skillet Meatloaf

Serves 4

Ingredients

- ❖ 2 1/2 lb. ground beef
- ❖ 1 small onion grated
- ❖ 1 garlic clove minced
- ❖ 1 egg
- ❖ 1 Tbsp. catsup
- ❖ Salt and pepper

Sauce:

- ❖ 1 can of tomato puree
- ❖ 1 tsp. sugar (omit or substitute with sweetener)
- ❖ Several fresh basil leaves chopped
- ❖ 1 small can of mushroom pieces drained
- ❖ 1 large onion sliced
- ❖ Worcestershire sauce

Direction

Make meatloaf mixture by combining meat, onion, egg and seasoning. Form into a round loaf.

Heat some olive oil in a heavy-duty skillet. Pat meat into pan and brown on both sides; carefully turning with wide spatula.

Mix tomato paste, an empty paste can of water, sugar and basil and pour over meatloaf. Add sliced onion and mushrooms to pan.

Sprinkle with a few splashes of Worcestershire sauce.

Cook covered over low heat for 1+ hour or until meatloaf is tender.

Occasionally stir sauce in pan and baste top of meatloaf. Serve meatloaf with some of the thickened sauce.

DIJON BEEF STEW

Ingredients

- ❖ 2 lb chuck stew meat
- ❖ 3 T olive oil
- ❖ 1/2 cup chopped onion
- ❖ 2 T soy flour or thickener
- ❖ 2 c beef broth
- ❖ 2 T dijon
- ❖ 1/2 lb mushrooms
- ❖ 1 T butter
- ❖ 1/4 c dry red wine

Direction

Dredge beef with flour. Saute in hot oil in Dutch oven. Add onions and cook til onions done and beef browned. Add broth and mustard. Simmer partially covered for 2-3 hours til meat tender.

Saute mushrooms in butter for 5 min and add wine. Bring to boil and add to stew. (Serves 4 @ 8 carb, 1 fiber (7 NET carbs), 666 Calories, 50 fat, 44 protein.

SALADS

Creamy Calico Salad

Serves 8

Ingredients

- ❖ 1 package lime sugar-free Jello
- ❖ 1 cup boiling water
- ❖ 1 cup cottage cheese
- ❖ ½ cup mayonnaise
- ❖ ½ cup heavy cream
- ❖ ¼ cup green onion, finely chopped
- ❖ ¼ cup red pepper, finely chopped
- ❖ ¼ cup celery, finely chopped
- ❖ ¼ cup carrot, grated

Direction

Place boiling water in blender container, add Jello. Let sit for a minute, then gently run blender to make sure it is fully dissolved. Add cottage cheese, cream, mayonnaise, and blend till smooth.

Mix in chopped vegetables and pour into a 4-cup jelly mould or bowl. Chill for at least four hours.

Dip mould into larger bowl filled with hot water for a second or two.

Unmould onto plate, decorate with red pepper strips. Serve and enjoy!

Notes: this can be made in a bowl if you like the cottage cheese in chunks. Any combination of chopped vegetables, even dill pickles or olives, that add up to 1 cup can be used, staying away from the more "liquid" types such as tomatoes or cucumber.

Total salad: 1,378 calories with 21.2 grams of carbohydrate

One serving: 172 calories with 2.7 grams of carbohydrate.

The Pantry Coleslaw

Ingredients

- ❖ 1 1/2 cups plus 2 tablespoons mayonnaise
- ❖ 6 tablespoons plus 1 teaspoon sugar (use artificial sweetener eqivilent)
- ❖ 3 tablespoons plus 1/2 teaspoon wine vinegar (optional)
- ❖ 1/2 to 3/4 cup oil
- ❖ 1/3 teaspoon each of garlic, onion, mustard, and celery powers
- ❖ Dash of black pepper
- ❖ 1 tablespoon plus 2 teaspoons of lemon juice (optional)
- ❖ 1 tablespoon plus 2 teaspoons half and half
- ❖ 1/2 teaspoon salt
- ❖ 2 heads cabbage, very finely shredded

Direction

Blend together mayonnaise, sugar, vinegar, and oil. Add spice powders, pepper, lemon juice, half and half and salt.

Stir until smooth. Pour over coleslaw in a large bowl and toss until cabbage is well coated. Dressing keeps well, covered tightly in the refrigerator for several days.

Makes 1 quart dressing.

Rare Roast Beef Salad with Mustard Mayonnaise

Serves 6

Dressing:

- ❖ 1/3 cup (3 1/2 fl oz/100 ml) olive oil
- ❖ 1/4 cup (2 fl oz/60 ml) lemon juice
- ❖ 2 tablespoons finely chopped chives
- ❖ 1 tablespoon drained tiny capers
- ❖ 1 tablespoon finely chopped sun-dried bell pepper
- ❖ Salt and freshly ground black pepper

Direction

Combine all dressing ingredients in a small bowl. Whisk together until well blended.

SOUPS

Gourmet Restaurant Cream of Almond Soup

Ingredients

- ❖ 6 c chicken stock
- ❖ 1/2 lb. ground toasted almonds
- ❖ 1/2 c heavy whipping cream
- ❖ 1/2 c water
- ❖ 4 egg yolks
- ❖ Salt and pepper to taste
- ❖ Chopped parsley
- ❖ Sliced almonds

Direction

Bring the stock to a boil. Add the almonds and simmer for fifteen minutes.

Beat together cream, water and the egg yolks. Whip the mixture into the stock and remove it from the heat.

Season to taste with salt and pepper. Garnish with chopped parsley and sliced almonds.

Curried Red Pepper Soup

Serves six as a first course

Ingredients

- ❖ 1 ½ pounds red, yellow, or orange sweet peppers (about 5-6)
- ❖ ½ cup chopped red onion
- ❖ 1 cup water
- ❖ 2 tsp. chicken bouillon granules
- ❖ 1 ½ tsp. curry powder or, to taste
- ❖ ½ tsp. dried thyme, crushed
- ❖ ½ tsp. dried marjoram, crushed
- ❖ 1 tsp. garlic powder
- ❖ 3 ounces cream cheese
- ❖ 1 2/3 cups whipping cream
- ❖ Sour cream (optional)

Direction

Halve peppers, seed, and remove internal membranes. Place on aluminium-foil covered cookie sheet and roast at 450 degrees for 10 - 15 minutes, until skins start to turn black and bubble.

Place in paper bag to steam and cool. When the peppers can be handled, remove skins and slice peppers into strips and place in a pan with onion, water, bouillon granules, curry powder, thyme, marjoram, and garlic. Simmer for 15 minutes. Add cream cheese cut into chunks. Puree mixture in blender or food processor until smooth. Stir in cream. To serve, swirl a teaspoon of sour cream on the top of each bowl.

Total calories - 1,351 Total grams carbohydrate - 46.1

Per serving - 226 calories 7.7 grams carbohydrate

Clam Chowder

Carbs: 4.33 per serving

Ingredients

- ❖ 1 stick butter
- ❖ 1 small onion, chopped
- ❖ 4 stalks celery, chopped
- ❖ 1 pint heavy cream
- ❖ 2 cans (16oz each) whole baby clams
- ❖ 1 cup clam broth
- ❖ 1/2 cup chicken broth (optional)
- ❖ 4 tablespoons thyme
- ❖ 4 tablespoons arrowroot
- ❖ 2 small tomatoes, chopped (optional)
- ❖ 8 spears asparagus, cut into 1/8ths
- ❖ Salt and pepper, to taste

Direction

In a medium size sauce pot, add the butter and melt on medium heat and sauté` till caramelized.

Now add the arrowroot, which will make a roue and thicken it a bit. Stir for 2-3 minutes.

Now, slowly add the heavy cream and stir well, making sure it does not come to a boil as the cream will burn. At this point, add the chicken broth - I used it, but not necessary) and lower the heat to a med-low setting. Add the clams, clam broth, tomatoes and asparagus, season with salt and pepper to taste, add more thyme if you like (I did).

VEGGIE

Company Peppers

Serves 6

Ingredients

- ❖ 1 each of red, orange, yellow and green sweet peppers 70 cals 10.1 carbs
- ❖ 2 tbsp. butter 204 cals 0.2 carbs
- ❖ 1 tsp. Splenda
- ❖ Salt and Pepper

<u>Direction</u>

Cut each pepper in half, remove seeds and internal ribs. Place on foil covered cookie sheet and roast in a 400-degree oven until pepper skin is bubbled and browned. Remove from oven, and place peppers in a paper bag to steam. When cool, remove skins and slice into long strips.

Sauté pepper strips in butter over medium/low heat for about 5 minutes (do not brown), adding Splenda, salt and freshly ground pepper.

This is a very colourful side dish and tastes as good as it looks.

Save leftovers with their liquid in fridge and throw into your next salad. Or puree with a little oil and vinegar for an outstanding pepper vinaigrette salad dressing.

Or reheat, add a tablespoon or so of cream, and serve over a portion of cooked spaghetti squash.

Total recipe: 276 calories, 10.8 grams of carbohydrate

Per serving: 46 calories, 1.8 grams of carbohydrate

Fauxtatoes

Ingredients

- ❖ 1 head cauliflower, chopped, cooked very soft
- ❖ 3 oz. cream cheese
- ❖ 1 tbsp. butter
- ❖ Salt and pepper to taste

<u>Direction</u>

Mash, whip with a mixer, or blend in food processor. Jamie adds.

"I've sometimes used a bag of frozen cauliflower, but I think a head of fresh cauliflower gives much better texture. I simmer the cauliflower with a chopped clove of garlic to cover mild "cabbage" taste."

Summer Squash Au-Gratin

Ingredients

2lbs summer squash

4 Tbsp. butter

1.5 Cups shredded cheddar

1 Cup sour cream

1/4 Cup chopped onion

1/3 cup parmesan cheese

Direction

Cook squash until tender. (I would cook only until slightly soft)
Drain well.

Mix with remaining ingredients and bake in casserole at 350
degrees for 20-30 minutes or until golden brown and bubbly.
Makes 6 servings.

Per serving: 311 calories, 26g fat (16 sat. fat), 70 Chol., 9g carb, 2g
fiber, 10g protein.

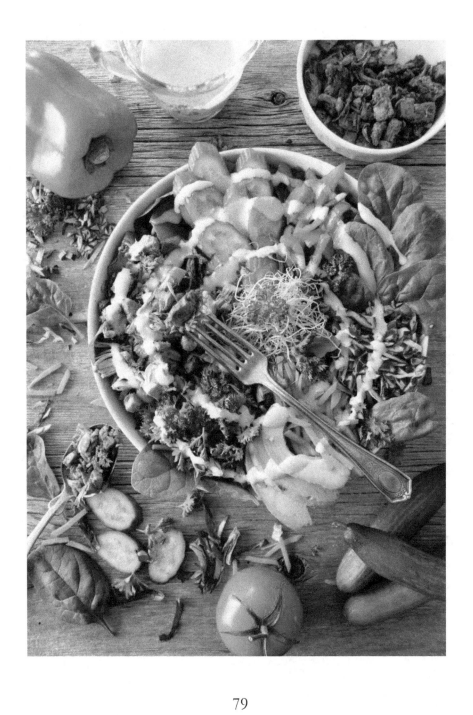

Becoming Vegetarian

It is always hard to accept and undergo changes; likewise altering to a vegetarian diet is not as easy as it may be presumed. So, it is very important to do an in-depth analysis before adapting to a new lifestyle. Sometimes, switching over to meatless diet might be difficult. Therefore, it is better to know the positive and negative effects beforehand, because becoming vegetarian involves a lot more than just cutting on meat.

There are several types of vegetarians like some who prefer eating fish and whereas some who do not. On the other hand, there are people who even do not consume dairy products including cheese and eggs and live on fruits and vegetables. Switching to vegetarian diet is always an individual's preference.

One must also keep in mind the nutritional supplements that body would require before you shun cottage cheese and other nutritional foods that provide essential nourishment.

It is better to start off slowly and progress gradually to be a total vegetarian. Though it is hard to believe, the entire body system will go through definite changes, since the body will not be getting something which it is very much habitual of. It is always better to reduce the quantity gradually, instead depriving meat from the routine diet suddenly, replace it by in-taking fish or chicken and then start cutting down the consumption gradually turning to be a total vegetarian.

The most important part in turning to a vegetarian style is to know the nutritional contents in the food which would be consumed instead of meat. Generally, those who do not approve of a vegetarian lifestyle, have an assumption that their body would be deprived of vital vitamins and minerals if meat is not added in the diet. Although, there are many who have been successful in switching over to a meatless diet. Such individuals have been able to supply their body with necessary nutrients and hence filling in the lag caused by the meatless diet.

Many researches have proved that the green vegetables like broccoli, kale and spinach contains enormous amounts of calcium and consumption of these green vegetables would give necessary nutrients to stay healthy.

As well, nuts are known to be rich source of protein. Consumption of such vegetarian diets can ensure that one gets enough to have a healthy life with balanced nutrition.

Turning to a vegetarian diet is one of the vital aspects that you can do to make your body feel healthy. And for individuals already converted to a vegan style, must have realized that they feel great and have excessive energy and were able lose weight without starving. So, start thinking on this and make a progress towards a satisfying lifestyle.

Cooking Gourmet Vegetarian

For individuals who are vegan and are fond of cooking gourmand dishes, there are enormous opportunities to explore and find.

There are a huge number of epicurean vegan recipes that an individual can cook in varied places and situations; you just need to seek prospects to do so. Regrettably, space limitation prevents us from enumerating a complete cookbook in this small article. But there are a few recommendations to offer regarding to tasty vegetarian food preparation.

Initially we begin by defining an epicure meal. Now the question arises that is this feasible? A gourmand meal is special meal devoid of meat or spaghetti and it includes converting interesting and rare elements into a masterpiece dishes that are not only delicious but also remarkable in appearance.

Evidently, gourmet can be explained by many people in many various ways but cooking a gourmet vegan food entails enough talent. It requires one to put a lot of flavour and ability to convert simple ingredients to artistic creations.

So, what must an individual know to cook a gourmand vegetarian meal? If they have been a lacto-vegetarian for rather some time, they might want to refer to ideas about what one likes to consume and how one can induce innovativeness to make it unusual and delicious as well as mouth-watering. If people are novel to vegetarian style of cooking, the best process is to bear in mind the type of gourmet meals they have had before. It is very true that almost each one of us has had vegetarian meals. One must always look out for ways one can shun out meat portion in the dish, while still maintaining intact the essence.

With a little mind and resourcefulness, this can be made possible - we know almost all can!

An individual can find enormous and diverse recipe books that are out-and-out devoted to gourmand vegetarian style of cooking in their local bookstore, on several web sites, and online. Surf for cooking methods that contain constituents that fascinate all and then try the recipe. Many will not be able to cook a gourmet vegetarian feast if they start from anywhere. But by stringently following the instructions, you can avert a gastronomic failure.

Cooking a gastronome meal can be a real adventurous and rejuvenating thing that a person ever does as a vegan chef. A lot of people believe the vegetarian way of life comprises of perplexity and inquisitiveness. When one can easily demonstrate that catering a vegetarian banquet that is epicurean, striking, and yummy, they may just wave them toward their side of the boundary.

But do not struggle very hard. Being a lacto-vegetarian is not for one and all. The finest things people can do is to cook with their heart and stay proper to their dedication of living a vegetarian style of living which signifies cooking foodie meals that savour like they have mutton when they do not have any meat content.

Eating Healthy Vegetarian

Vegan diets are known to be very hale and hearty but eating a reasonable food when an individual is a vegetarian, it usually attracts little additional notice. When a person shuns red meat and animal protein out of their diet, they are shunning out a chief resource of protein which their body requires.

It means that eating healthy diet as a vegan will entail adding foods into one's diet that will endow with nutrients commonly found in meat foodstuffs.

By exploring a diet consisting of fruits, vegetables, and whole grains, people can easily avail vitamins and nutrients they want from vegetarian sources so that their vegetarian way of life is healthy and in proportion.

By consuming food items like legumes, soy foods, nuts, and eggs, one can obtain the essential protein content that they require to nurture. One must also keep in mind that other nutrients like the minerals iron, calcium, and the vitamins D and B12, are equally vital for vegans.

Whereas it is factual that removing meat out of one's diet and consuming a diet rich in vegetables, fruits, and grains is healthy. But vegetarians require worrying about other things essential nutrients like receiving the right balance of vitamins and minerals from their diet.

Many can constantly take a vitamin add-on, but since a lot of these supplements include animal derivatives, many devoted vegetarians hesitate in taking them. It is essential that one must look out for a diet which is rich in vitamins B and C, iron and niacin since they are also vital part of a healthy lacto-vegetarian way of life.

A person does not have to forgo one's health when they prefer to become a vegan. Ingestion of healthy vegetarian diet is not an easy task. One must exclusively take leisure time to study and find food items that include nutrients most essential for the body. For this, perhaps you will have to go extensively through several books, magazines or even surf internet.

People can make all kinds of swaps in their diet that can replace meat when are not eating any longer. For instance, one can opt for soy milk as an alternative to cow's milk which in turn will provide the necessary calcium to the body.

Including nuts and grains into a vegetarian diet suitably turns it into a healthy diet. Also, nuts and grains are full of proteins which are helpful in developing healthy bones.

Several Studies have revealed that vegetarians generally have healthy eating routine that leads to a fit and healthy body. They also have a higher tendency to remain healthy and energetic.

The thing people need to keep in mind for healthy vegan diet is that they must give particular interest to nutrient content present in the foods that they eat and be sure to eat balanced diet.

How to Become a Vegetarian

It may possibly seem impractical to imagine the initiatives a person should take to study to turn to a vegetarian diet. Nevertheless, it is not as simple as merely hacking meat out of one's diet?

The response to that straightforward issue is.... not actually.

People perceive that becoming a vegan requires much more effort, than simply refusing to a steak or a hamburger. An individual would discover that exploring to become a vegan entails a lot of examination and some serious efforts, so that one can be fit and not devoid their body of something that it essentially requires to function completely in the manner it was intended to.

The most important thing one requires to attempt when turning to a vegan diet is to take it leisurely. If you have been habitual of consuming meat for years now, in that case a laid-back attitude will not make much difference.

You will have to make some serious and planned efforts to become a vegan. Begin by slashing meat out of your regular diet gradually. You can cut on meat for some days and then switch over to consuming fish or chicken.

This process can eventually help you in quitting meat permanently as the body slowly and progressively gets used change in diet. If an individual desires to realize how to adopt a lacta-vegetarian diet, then they will also have to do petite exploration into the nutrients that are comprised in different vegetables, so a person can be certain that their body is receiving the essential stuff it requires to be well-built as well as efficient. It must be kept in mind that vitamins like B and C as well as minerals like iron and zinc are essential for the human.

Calcium and protein are also vital components of a proportionate diet, so one would wish to know the nutritional value of the food that they are consuming. It is necessary to ensure that the body is provided all the essential nutrients and vitamins that it requires to function efficiently. Because people are removing meat from their diet, they must ensure that they intake sufficient protein into their body. Protein is crucial for human body and hence when people are studying how to turn into a vegan, they desire to get substitute supplies of protein.

Low Calorie Vegetarian Recipes

Maybe an individual would have preferred a vegetarian standard of living because they wish to drop weight and require low calorie vegan approach to aid them in their weight loss objectives.

The excellent news is that merely by changing over to meat free eating; one would be ingesting low calories. The unrevealed aspect of preparing healthy vegan recipes is to remove additional flab that makes meals filling.

Initially, when a person is preparing low-fat vegan recipes, people will want to avoid the use of too much oil. An individual can yet use a superior quality additional virgin olive oil for tastings and salads.

EVOO has less caloric value and gives some of "beneficial fats" that our body need. Discourage fried foods while you are preparing vegetarian recipes which are less in caloric value. Even if one does use added virgin olive oil for frying, despite this, fried foods characteristically have higher calories, so one should shun fried foods as much as feasible.

Steam the vegetables as an alternative and refrain from boiling them. Boiling will deplete significant nutrients. Grill vegetables for some change.

You can also apply a no calorie or light cooking spray to provide them some wetness or even scatter on a little watery lemon juice.

If one's diet permits them to eat seafood, boil fish despite frying it. It is advisable to grill the fish since grilling is an immense mode to add taste and distinctiveness to their foods. Spices are main ingredients that can bring a vast change and provide a low-fat vegetarian recipe that is enjoyable and yummy.

A lot of recipes of low-calorie vegetarian dishes can be found online. An individual can also purchase vegetarian cookery books with low-fat recipes in them.

A more practical and an effortless method for making low calorie vegetarian recipes is to just alter usual recipes by using healthy replacements like diet cheeses or replacing plain yogurt for vinegary cream. If an individual is creative, they will be amazed to discover that you can discover plenteous healthy vegetarian recipes and able utilize these recipes into one's diet that will balance their weight loss targets.

All a person requires is a little learning into where one can make replacements that will turn high calorie foods into light foods with a small amount of variation and numerous thoughts. Embrace low calorie vegan recipes into your daily diet plan, become conscious that you can consume tasty foods while sustaining your meatless standard of living.

Low Carb Vegetarian

Human bodies need various nutrients to stay fit. Being vegetarian is good, but you need to balance the vitamins and nutrients skilfully. The only thing that should come in your mind is the balance of carbs. Carbs are a great source of energy and that is the only reason to consume carbs in proper proportion. Excess of carbs in a vegetarian diet will trigger fat production in human body. Carbs alter sugar which in turn changes into fat and this creates problem if the quantity of conversion is in excess.

Some foods are rich in carbohydrates like rice, potato and grains, so if you have plans to low down on carb intake, you should minimize the consumption of such foods. It is also not advisable to completely cut these foods in your diet as these are good source of carbs. Efforts should be done to curtail the consumption of these food products.

Carbs are also present in flour which also includes the whole wheat flour. You should avoid or minimize eating bread if you are serious about the proper carbs intake. Make sure, that the source of your carbs is appropriate to control the suitable consumption of carbs.

Stay away from white bread and eat whole grain bread to compensate the carb requirement of body.

Being vegetarian is good, but you must give up lot of things during the process. Diet should include a lot of fresh, green vegetables.

Selection of oils for preparing the food should also be considered. If you are using olive oil you must use the proper quantity to reach the required level of carb. Also consider steaming and grilling of oil to ensure low carb intake. You have the natural vitamins in green and leafy vegetables. Do not consume carbohydrates that will make you gain weight.

Different people have different reasons for changing their lifestyle to a vegetarian one. The most basic reason is losing extra weight. Some people also are really concerned about killing of various animals. A well-balanced diet is the most important criteria behind a vegetarian lifestyle. Excess amount of carbohydrates can change into sugar which can gradually lead to gaining extra weight.

Before you follow a vegetarian diet that is also low in carbohydrate content, you must be very careful in finding the exact amount of carbohydrate present in your diet. If the amount of carbs is very low, then it may affect your body and most importantly your health. The most important part of a healthy diet is nutrition.

Low Fat Vegetarian Eating

Everyone knows that once you continue with diet devoid of meat, you are assured of low-fat intake. In this way the article title is a bit oxymoron because vegetable diet is out of fat-based products. A question arises as to why we should give this title low fat vegetarian eating. Since fats are also necessary for body to function properly, emphasis should be given on natural fat-based products. Eating healthy and keeping your fat levels low can be obtained by vegetarianism as well. When natural fats come into picture you should try and accommodate right proportion of fat in your diet.

There are many sources of fat-based diets. Fishes have the best fat-based elements known as Omega 3 fatty acids. Such fatty acids give us controlled amount of fat that is required by the human body to stay fit. The problem comes when you decide to be vegan and not a vegetarian because vegans do not eat fish. Whet will be the source of fats?

This question keeps hunting people who wants to follow vegan type of food group.

Leaving meats and fishes you can derive fats from other products as well. Extra virgin olive oil, which is also known as EVOO, has fats that are very good for our system. Low fats are always good and work excellent with vegetarians. You should not take this olive oil in excess if you are vegetarian. Proper proportion should be taken to fulfil the fat requirement of the body. Flax seed and oils from flax seeds should be tried to compensate the fat requirement of vegetarians. Nuts cooked with a good amount of pine nuts are also good source of fats for vegetarians. Peanuts are suggested by many experts to make your diet complete.

The best food to substitute fats in the body is cheese. In case if you are vegetarian, then it is advisable to make cheese an essential part of your diet plan as you have embraced dairy food items and eggs. Cheese stands to be one of the finest suited options for diets rich in fats. People belonging to Wisconsin have a natural tendency to intake cheese. The major aspect to keep in mind is that you must opt for good cheese and add it as an essential item of your vegetarian diet. But, the amount of cheese intake must be checked cautiously, since it tastes good but an overwhelming serving of cheese on regular basis can harm your body.

Vegetarian diet includes low fat intake and consuming a total vegan diet is like naturally eating foods low in fat content. You must check on what kind of food you should eat and what to avoid. To conclude a proper mix of all the nutrients and vitamins will form a healthier and a disease-free system.

This will also provide you a slimmer body, healthy lifestyle, and an excellent way of living.

Vegan Vegetarian

The difference between vegetarian and non-vegetarian is widely understood as the eating habits are distinct and obvious. There is another branch of food eating group commonly known as vegan and difference between vegetarian and vegan is misunderstood.

There is no striking difference between vegan and vegetarian eating habits but still people get confused in categorizing these food eating groups. As a layman you will not be able to understand the difference between vegan and vegetarian.

People consider these as same food eating groups because the similarities are obvious and clear.

People believe what they see, and you often spot a vegetarian eating green fresh salads and few broccolis for all three meals. The fact is different vegans and vegetarians consume foods very differently and their ways are not always similar. Understanding the eating trends of this faction will make things clear. Below are few examples.

People who consume dairy products, eggs, fruits, and vegetables are categorized as Lacto-ovo-vegetarian. It is one of the most recurrent and frequent type of lacto-vegetarian diet. There are cases where you find these groups eating fish and consuming poultry products.

Lacto-vegetarian: Their diet includes vegetables, healthy nuts, fruits, grains and dairy products. The only difference is egg consumption which this group avoids.

Vegan: The difference between vegans and vegetarian can be understood by following their food habits. Vegans do not include dairy foodstuffs, eggs or any sort of animal products in their regular diet. Not only have these vegans refrained from sporting or wearing anything which is derived from animal products.

Macrobiotic: There are many reasons to follow a diet group. Diet which is followed on grounds of philosophy and spirituality is known as Macrobiotic diet. Health factors are also considered before selecting this diet. In this diet food is categorized as negative and positive food. The positive group is the ying and negative is yang. There are levels of progression in this type of diet. The elimination of animal products is encouraged at all levels. The highest level eliminates even fruits and vegetables and is confined to brown rice.

A normal person will get confused between the lacto-vegetarian and vegetarian diet. But for vegans and vegetarian it is easy to follow their lifestyle.

It is only when you start to follow a diet regime you come to know the positives and negatives. You should support all diet groups and food eating habits as far as it's healthy and keeps you strong.

Vegetarian Cooking for Everyone

Cooking vegetarian food is indeed one of the easiest things to learn. Even those who fear boiling water or cooking dishes will find vegetarian food very interesting and easy to prepare. Vegetarian cooking is for everyone. It not only has high nutritional value, but also vegetarian cooking is easy for everyone.

Deborah Madison, America's top chef just recently came out with his bestseller book 'Vegetarian Cooking for Everyone'. One must not think of it as just another vegetarian cooking book. It has some delicious 800 recipes and vital answers to questions about components and procedures of cooking. One can learn new way to cook some known dishes like Guacamole from the book and even some lesser-known ones like Green Lentils with Roasted Beets and Preserved Lemons, and Cashew Curry.

For all its readers it has proved to be a great source book and has ensured a great learning experience. In fact, one of the readers confessed that the author is writing recipes for everyday kitchen and this is what attracts readers from all age groups. It is not liked those chef books which the reader or a learner feels difficult to prepare. 'Vegetarian Cooking for Everyone' is a book for everyone. An average cook can even cook or prepare good dishes reading from it. For a new learner or beginner this is of great help who can feel his confidence being lifted when he can prepare good vegetarian dishes that taste delicious.

'Vegetarian Cooking for Everyone' has been adjudged as a comprehensive book that is of interest to all, even those who want to seek its help in everyday cooking as well. It has recipes for all starting from starters, sizzlers, snacks breakfast lunch and dinner. The ingredients are simple and can be easily found in one's fridge and pantry and cook something great out of it all which is a huge satisfaction and a source of joy.

Vegetarian Cooking

There is a different method of cooking for a vegetarian lifestyle. You can also find out the nutritional value in your diet. Many people may not find vegetarian cooking as interesting as the non-vegetarian cooking. There are different methods and styles of preparing vegetarian food as well. All the various means will hence increase your interest in the vegetarian preparation. The simple thought of vegetarian cooking can thus make cooking interesting.

You can find versatility in vegetarian foods. You can also prepare them in several different ways. The best example is to slice up an eggplant into thick portions of about an inch. Then you can make it more creative by layering them with parmesan and ricotta. Special use of mozzarella cheese for vegetarian lasagne is the best example.

Take egg plant and add a small number of breadcrumbs to it and always fry it in olive oil. Olive oil has less fat containing elements and that is good for health as well.

Green salad should be consumed because it has great nutritional value. The level of nutrition you can get from vegetarian food will have the capacity to suffice your requirements. Egg burgers should also be tried as a part of vegetarian diet. The protein part from eggs gives lot of strength to the body.

Usage of spices should be given emphasis because spices can make or break the taste. After the dish is prepared you should try and sprinkle some asparagus to add more taste to the dish. You can try butter spray to get an amazing taste. If you want to experience some tangy twist you can try spritz broccoli which is steamed with a dash of lemon juice to add flavour.

You must think outside the box if you want to do some vegetarian cooking. There are exciting ways to make things interesting.

Cooking needs a lot of innovation and great cooks of the world believe that there are ten thousand unique dishes that can be prepared by using all the vegetables available in the world.

The treatment of tomato can do wonders. Tomato is an excellent vegetable, and you can experiment many different dishes by using tomatoes. If you like cheese, then you can top the tomato with different kind of cheese to add taste to the preparation. Tomato gives unique and defined taste to any vegetarian dish. You can innovate several types of dishes by using tomatoes. When you have so many options open by using a single vegetable imagine range of varieties if you explore more vegetables.

Just utilize your creative instincts and you can create wonders with vegetables. Once you become a vegetarian you will fall in love with the vegetables. Living with fewer options is not advisable because you will get bored of eating same dish again and again. Meatless options can make you forget meat. When you have researched well and explored options then you will encourage vegetarianism.

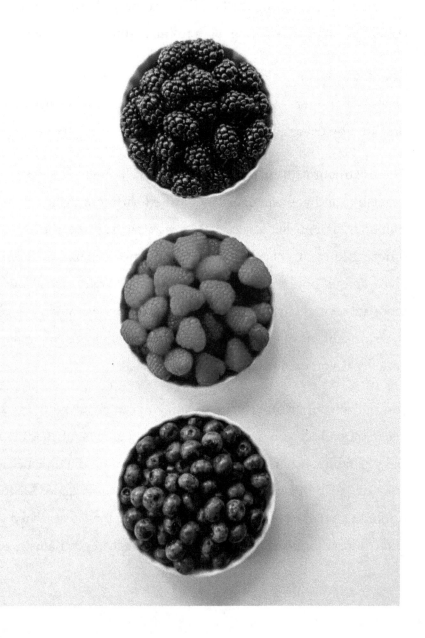

CPSIA information can be obtained
at www.ICGtesting.com
Printed in the USA
BVHW091020300421
605944BV00027B/747